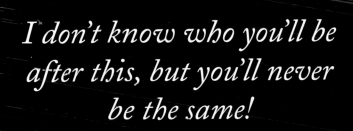

I don't know who you'll be after this, but you'll never be the same!

JOIN US.
JOIN THE WAR.

You've dieted before.

You've lost weight then gained it all back.

Today that ends.

Hold yourself accountable and we will battle

with you every step of the way.

SIGN HERE TO JOIN THE WAR:

_____

*Share this page with the world.

Take a picture and share it on your social media pages.

Let everyone know you have joined the War on Carbs!

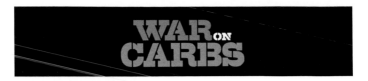

TABLE OF CONTENTS

THE LOW-DOWN

THE DIET

THE DETAILS

1. INTRODUCTION

I have found a diet that works really well for me. It doesn't require me to weigh my food, pee on a stick, count calories, or prick my finger. And losing body fat is the result.

My first stint with a ketogenic-style diet was in 1995 because of a guy named Ron Fedkiw. I was preparing for a powerlifting meet, and I wanted to get down to the next weight class, which at the time was 198 lbs. About two weeks prior to the competition, I decided, on my own, to start a bodybuilding-style diet to lose the weight—high protein, high carb, low fat.

I was talking to my brother and told him what I was doing. He said, "No, no, no. You need to talk to my friend Ron." And I said, "What does Ron do?" He said that Ron has a Ph.D. in Mathematics. And I said, "What does that have to do with my dieting for a powerlifting meet?" He said, "Just give the guy a call. Trust me. He knows what he's talking about."

So I called him up, and he said, "Your brother told me the asinine shit you were going to do to lose weight for your powerlifting meet, but here's what you need to do. Do you have a pen?" I said, "Nope." He said, "Do you have a piece of paper?" I said, "Nope." Of course, as usual, I could not find either one for a very long time. After I got my shit together, I said, "I'm ready."

He replied with, "Okay, here's the diet. Red meat. Water. Salt. Period ."

Guess what? I not only made weight, I won the contest, I made the lifts, and I performed well. That was my introduction to a keto-style diet.

After the contest, I remember thinking, "Holy shit, that diet really changed the way I looked very quickly." From that point on, while other people were eating sandwiches from the local deli, I was eating mounds of meat and cheese.

2. ME: BEFORE AND AFTER

Then

This is me before.
This is what I used to do.
This is what I used to eat.
This is what I used to look like.

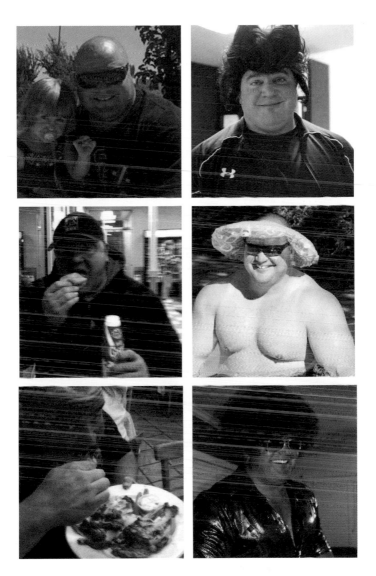

Now

This is me.
This is what I do now.
This is what I eat now.
This is what I look like now.

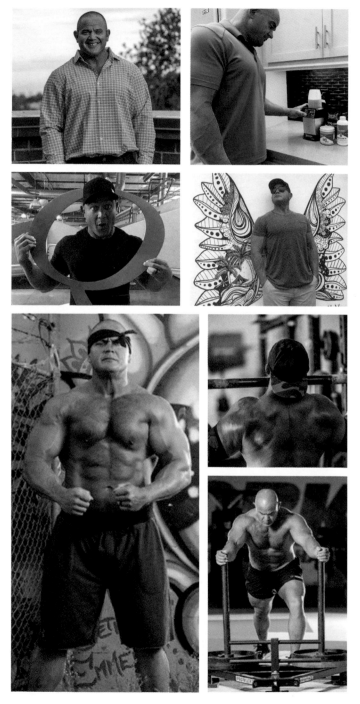

"STRENGTH IS NEVER A WEAKNESS."

3. WHO ARE YOU?

I receive a lot of questions about motivation. As a coach, I've heard it all: people say they've become injured or sick. They got thrown off course. They got married. All kinds of weird shit happens to you, right? Life happens, and life can definitely interfere with some of the things we love to do. The reason why I never stop is because I'm always thinking: WHO AM I? Think about that for a minute: Who Are You? Who Are YOU? Who the Hell Are You?

Are you the person your parents named you after?
Are you that name?
Do you represent that name?

WHO ARE YOU?

Who you are is not determined by who you want to be. It's determined by people's perception of you. Our perception is our reality. How do people perceive you? Nobody's full blast, nobody's full bore 24 hours a day, 7 days a week. We all have our shortcomings.

I am a lifter. When I step into the gym, I'm trying to bring it every single time. I'm not a tough guy, I'm no special person. If I were a tough guy, I'd be fighting in the UFC. But I'm not. That's not me. That's not what I do. I'm a lifter. And you've got to think, what's the perception of you out there? So if you lose motivation, if you've fallen off the wagon and shit starts falling apart, start thinking about that for a minute. Start thinking about not only what other people are going to think of you, but also how you're going to think of yourself.

If you're lazy, you're not stepping up, and you're not putting in your time, that'll be the word that's going around about you.

I've put a lot of time into the gym, as many of you have. I've had my moments where I've done well, and I've had my moments where I've done shitty. At times, I'm very motivated, and at times I'm not. You're not always going to be 100% motivated to go kick some ass. So how do you stay motivated? How do you stay fired up?

One of the best ways to become the best YOU is to set goals for yourself that are within reach to be successful. Don't say you want to squat 1,000 lbs. when you haven't squatted 700 yet. Don't be delusional. Tell yourself, "You know what? I want to squat 720 lbs." Or, "I want to feel 800 lbs. in the gym. I just want to un-rack it." Set small goals for yourself now, so when you accomplish them, they build on themselves. Success breeds success. For every successful moment you have, you can think of it as a giant pat on the back. And every time you get a pat on the back, it's giving you more and more confidence. That confidence will build and build and build and when you're that confident it's a little bit easier to stay motivated. When you get down on yourself, that's when things start to get a little harder. So keep your chin up, keep training hard. And remember that part of knowing who you are is knowing who you are not. Work on figuring that shit out. But in the meantime, get your ass in the gym and train hard.

4. HOW THE WAR ON CARBS CAME TO BE

It was August 2016. My brother and I were at a sushi restaurant in Davis, CA. As we were sitting there he said, "You know what, I'm just too damn fat." I agreed with him. I said, "Yes, indeed. You are too fat." He said, "I need to do something big. I need to make a big change." And I said, "How about from here to the Olympia (which was about three weeks away) let's not eat any more carbs."

As we sat there with piles of rice in front of us, my brother said, "Yeah, fuck carbs!" I said, "Yeah, it's us versus them!" Then he shouted out with excitement, "This is a War on Carbs!"

We joined forces right there on the spot, the way William Wallace does in Braveheart when he unites the clans — with a good old-fashioned, manly, forearm handshake.

At the time, we didn't realize what this would become or that I was going to write a book about it, or that while I was writing this book I would be in the process of filming a documentary about it. In the last year, this diet has knocked off more than 100 lbs. total from both my brother and me.

This diet has also evaporated pounds from thousands of our fans from around the globe . We have battled together, and we are looking for more soldiers in this War on Carbs. So without further ado, join us as we start the War on Carbs.

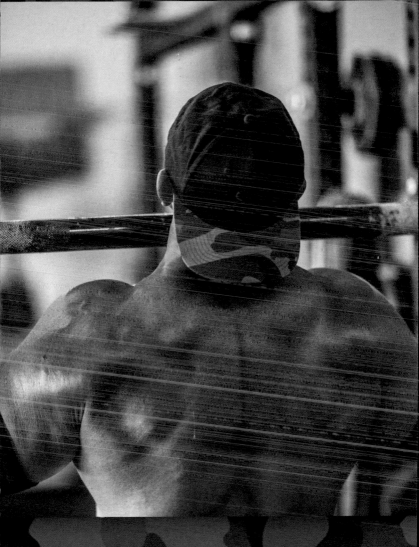

5. WHAT THE HELL IS IT?

The War on Carbs is a no-carb, no-bullshit diet that shifts the body from using carbohydrates as its main energy source to using fat. This is known as a ketogenic-style diet.

What is a Ketone? A ketone is produced when the body metabolizes or breaks down fat. Your body is then able to use the ketones as fuel to power everyday functions.

I'm not big on percentages or numbers. I do not count calories, and I do not count my percentages of fat or protein or any of that, but here are some recommended numbers:

MY RECOMMENDED PERCENTAGES
FOR DAILY MACROS:
60-90% Fat
20-30% Protein
0-10% Carbohydrates

In order to get your specific macros, you can check out a Keto Calculator online. Here's one we like: ruled.me/keto-calculator

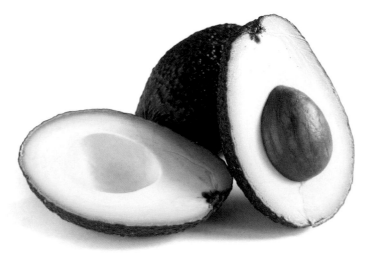

"BE MADE OF SOMETHING DIFFERENT."

6.   THE DIET

With many best-selling diet books, it's hard to even find the actual diet in the book. This book, the War on Carbs, is different… and in my opinion — way better! So here it is.

THE WAR ON CARBS DIET PLAN

WHAT TO EAT:
Fat
Protein
Vegetables

WHAT TO AVOID:
Carbohydrates

If you're like me, and you don't like to read diet books, here's what you're going to be eating for the next 14 days:

PROTEINS:
• Red meat
• Chicken (the fatty parts – or with skin on it)
• Pork
• Fish
• Eggs
• Cheese
• Cured meats, such as salami, pepperoni, etc.

FATS:
• Nuts
• Avocados
• Olives
• Olive oil
• MCT oil/coconut oil
• Butter
• Fish oil
• Ghee
• Cheese

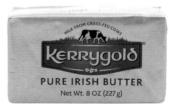

CARBS:
• Vegetables

BEVERAGES:
• Coffee
• Water
• Unsweetened Tea

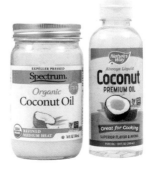

HERE'S WHAT I ACTUALLY EAT:
FOR PROTEIN:
• Steak – filet mignon, rib eye, New York strip, and prime rib
• Hamburger patties
• Pork – this means bacon!
• Fish – I like salmon best!
• Chicken – I eat the thighs and the drums. Eat the skin, too. Don't be a chicken.
• Cheese of any kind

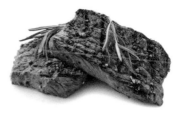

FOR FATS:
• Nuts! Almonds are my favorite but you can eat any kind of nuts you like.
• Avocados – Mmm
• Butter
• Heavy cream
• Half and half
• Olive oil
• Avocado oil
• Macadamia nut oil
• Coconut oil rich in MCT
• MCT Oil – MCTs convert to ketones and provide energy fast.

FOR VEGGIES:
• Any and all are fine and I'd suggest at least two servings a day prepared any way you want.

THINGS I DON'T EAT (WHILE ON THE WAR ON CARBS):
• Carbs in general
• Sugar – Check the labels, sugar is in everything.
• Rice
• Potatoes
• Fruit
• Cookies
• Pizza
• Ice Cream
• And anything else that tastes good #kidding #notreallykidding

TIPS:
• Drink lots of water
• Add a dash or two of salt to some meals
• Cut out sugar
• Keep your trace carbs as low as you can with the foods above.
(Trace means less than 1 g, so a food label can say
0 g of carbs, but it may still contain up to 1 g of carbs per serving.
These can add up quickly.)

EXAMPLES OF NUMBERS FOR DIFFERENT BODY WEIGHTS:
• A 200 lb. guy would need about 200 grams of fat, 200 grams of
protein, and as little carbs as possible. To find your specific numbers,
use a keto calculator! There are plenty online. Just search "Keto Calculator." And keep in mind that we might have to manipulate these
numbers based on your intended result.

Wham! That's the easy part. Now, read on if you want to know why
it works.

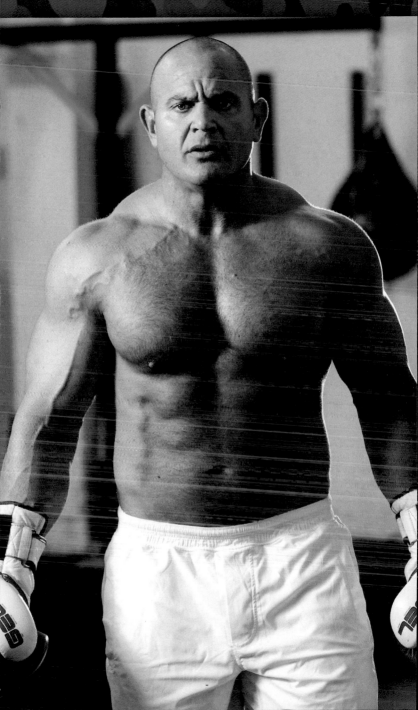

7.   WHAT IS KETOSIS?
WHAT ARE KETONES?

Ketosis: a normal metabolic process. It occurs when the body does not have enough glucose for energy and it burns stored fats instead. This results in a build-up of acids called ketones within the body. Some people encourage ketosis by following a diet called the ketogenic or low-carb/high-fat diet. People also prefer to get into ketosis for mental clarity and to lose weight.

Ketone: I consider the ketone a "fourth macronutrient," and our bodies use it as an energy source when carbohydrates are absent[1]. In terms of this book, "keto" means we're on a diet that is low enough in carbs and high enough in fat that it allows our bodies to produce ketones.

[1] Lowery PHD, Ryan, Wilson, Dr. J. (2017). The Ketogenic Bible: The Authoritative Guide to Ketosis. Canada: Victoria Belt Publishing Inc.

"YOU'RE EITHER IN OR YOU'RE IN THE WAY."

8. HOW THIS DIET CAN BENEFIT YOU

I feel this diet can help millions of people, but I'm also smart enough to understand that it's possible that it doesn't fit everyone's needs. That's just life. One thing this diet does do (that in my opinion a lot of other diets don't do) is walk you through levels of discipline that are not addressed on other diets.

When it comes to counting calories or flexible dieting, which are almost the same thing, they give you too much leeway to fall back into bad habits.

In order to change your body, you have to change your mind. Hey, you should write that down!

In order for this to work, we need to be focused on the small goals first.

When we exercise discipline over and over again, it tends to build success. And the more success you have, the better you'll feel. Eventually, those good feelings toward having stronger discipline will turn into what is called a pattern. In my opinion, by shutting off the impulse of eating carbs, it's easier to stay on course.

I've done and tried, utilized and experimented with just about every diet out there. I've read The Zone Diet, The Anabolic Diet, The Body Opus, The Bulletproof Diet, and The Paleo Solution. I learned a lot over the years and developed my own opinions. In the end, I always returned to the low-carb style of diet. The real magic of this diet is that it helps you create new patterns.

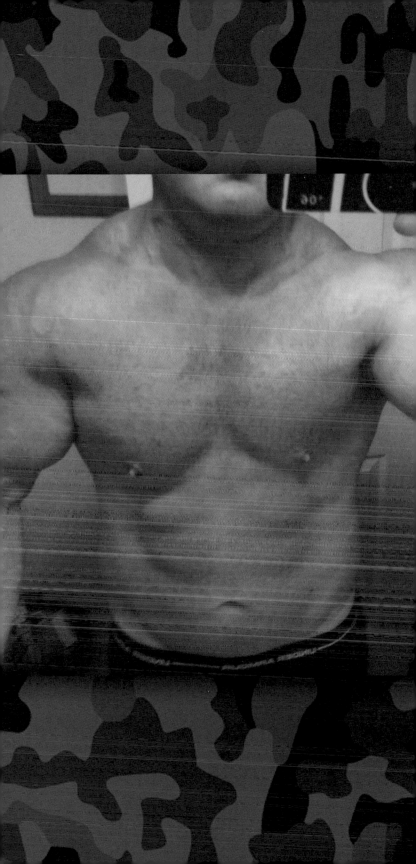

9.   GETTING STARTED

KEYS TO SUCCESS

Here are a few good rules that will help you get started on the War on Carbs:

1. Don't reduce calories. There's no good reason to go full keto and reduce calories at the same time. Our goal is food first—think about the food we need that will help us get into ketosis. This process is going to take about two weeks or more depending on the person.
2. Don't fast. We're not implementing fasting yet. This is something we'll talk about later. If you're experienced with keto and fasting, then proceed with doing whatever you feel is going to be best for you. But reducing calories, going keto, and fasting would be a huge shock and could leave you with negative feedback.
3. Don't allow yourself to get too hungry. Always have keto snacks on hand.
4. Don't eat carbs. Don't eat carbs. Just don't eat carbs.

THINGS TO HAVE

You don't have to buy a bunch of stuff to be on this diet, but here are a few things that can help get you going in the right direction immediately.

IN YOUR PANTRY:
• C-8 MCT oil
• Avocado oil
• Olive oil
• Grass-fed butter (grass-fed products have better fat and amino acid profiles)
• Eggs
• Bacon
• 80/20 grass-fed hamburger meat
• Cheese – any cheese will do, but Tillamook® Medium Cheddar Natural Cheese is my favorite for flavor and fat profile
• Raw almonds
• Cashews
• Macadamia nuts
• Raw walnuts
• Vegetables
• Cured meats

There is a lot more food on the diet, but these are some quick simple things that you can buy online (or at your local store) to get started right away.

AT WORK OR ON-THE-GO:

It's ok to start with small changes.

• If you eat out, order a burger without the bun or a sandwich without the roll.

• If you're going to the movies or going to work, bring keto snacks with you so you're not tempted to eat off the diet.

If you're not preparing to succeed, then you're preparing to fail. We need to constantly set ourselves up for success. Going on vacation or travelling for work is not an excuse to go off the diet. If you stay prepared, and don't allow yourself to get too hungry, you can continually make good decisions and go around the corners rather than cut them. These are keto snacks that should always be on-hand:

• Duke's Sausages®
• Tillamook® cheese squares
• Cheese sticks
• Nuts
• Hard boiled eggs (can also be found at grocery stores, at the airport, and even Starbucks)
• Cured meats – salami, pepperoni, etc.
• Keto Bars
• Keto Kookie
• Phat Fudge

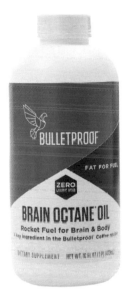

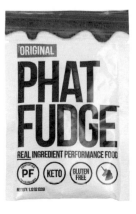

10. THREE PHASES OF THE WAR ON CARBS

Think of these as steps. Complete one phase before moving on to the next.

PHASE ONE

War on Carbs: No cheat day. We're trying to go as many days as possible without carbs. Just so you don't get the wrong idea, this isn't a contest and you're not trying to go the rest of your life without carbs. However, you need to take the stance to make some big changes and commit to something harder and stronger than you ever have before. Set goals for yourself. Can you go 10 days? How about 20 days? See if you can go 30 or 40 days. Choosing an enormous amount time isn't going to ensure that you're going to have rapid weight loss, but the longer you can go, the better.

The longer you go, the more you will begin to develop a stronger mindset and stronger thought patterns. The result of a stronger mindset will be your ability to develop better habits.

Once you're in ketosis, which may take a few days to a few months depending on the person, you may want to implement fasting. Try a 12-hour fast (no food, only water or black coffee), a 16-hour fast, or an 18-hour fast. Fasting will help boost your ketone levels. Once you've been fighting the War on Carbs for 2-3 months, you're ready to move on to Phase two.

PHASE TWO

Cyclical Ketogenic-style Diet. There are many other diets that are similar to this, such as The Anabolic Diet by Dr. Mauro DiPasquale[2], The Carb Nite Solution by John Kiefer[3], and the Body Opus Diet by Dan Duchaine[4]. Phase two of this diet allows for a cheat window of 4-6 hours one time per week.

Naturally, your first thought is going to be to throw down a pint of ice cream, or a bag of peanut butter cups, but by this time you're probably worried about what's going to happen to your stomach after not eating this way for so many weeks. My suggestion to kick off this cheat window would be to have a healthy meal that is just kind of normal and digests okay. For example, go out to sushi and eat the rice. Or go to a teriyaki chicken place and eat a rice bowl or a burrito. Once you've done that and rested or recuperated, then you can finish your night off with some sweets or real junk. I do not recommend turning this into an eating contest that leaves you bloated and in tons of pain and has you sitting on the toilet the whole next day. However, if that's what happens then screw it! It's okay because the next day, we're getting right back on the plan.

I refer to the day after a cheat meal as a "food hangover." Usually, the best thing for a hangover is the drug that got you there in the first place. But we are going to steer back on course and forbid ourselves to eat junk food. We're going to use exercise. And, we are going to eat some War on Carbs staple foods to get us back on track.

Once you graduate from Phase two, you can move on.

PHASE THREE
Performance Enhancing Diet—PED. This phase allows for more carbohydrates. Carbs are to be eaten before and after training sessions only. On a typical training day, you might be upwards of 100-150 gram of carbs, which includes your post-workout OJ + Gatorade cocktail, and 30-60 grams on non-training days. Note: If you try one of these phases, you may find yourself falling back into the same pitfalls and you might have a carb relapse. If you find yourself getting out of rhythm with your diet, revert back to the War on Carbs Phase One.

[2]DiPasquale, Dr. M. (1995). The Anabolic Diet. Optimum Training Systems.

[3]Kiefer, J. (2005). The Carb Nite Solution: The Physicist's Guide to Power Dieting. Charleston, SC: BookSurge Publishing

[4]Duchaine, D. (1996). Underground Bodyopus: Militant Weight Loss & Recomposition. XIPE Press.

11. WAR ON CARBS
A TYPICAL DAY

WITH A COFFEE FAST

My "coffee fast" could also be used as a fat fast because I add butter and MCT oil to my coffee. However, a coffee fast can also refer to when you only drink black coffee with nothing in it. On the other hand, a fat fast is when you're only consuming fats while you're fasting. So, you can do a coffee fast that's just coffee, without fat. And that is a coffee fast. Or you can do a coffee fast and use it as a fat fast as well. I call my coffee fast a fat fast because the percentage of fat is through the roof. It's primarily just fat. It should also be noted that my schedule never has me eating past 9 p.m.

5:30 a.m. – Coffee + butter + Keto Pro + MCT Oil
12ish – Steak + eggs
2:30 p.m. – Lifting
6 p.m. – Sushi, without the rice of course. Japanese people call this sashimi. I have a salad with it.
9 p.m. – 1 scoop of Keto Pro + peanut butter + heavy whipping cream + cinnamon

SUPPLEMENTS

I take most of my supplements with that last meal before bed. And I drink a lot of water because I take a lot of pills. Consult with your physician to help you choose what supplements will most likely be a good fit for you.

"THE ROAD TO NOWHERE IS PAVED WITH EXCUSES."

12. CYCLICAL KETOGENIC-STYLE DIET A TYPICAL DAY

See "War on Carbs – a typical day" but add a cheat meal once a week. See section about cheat days to keep yourself in check.

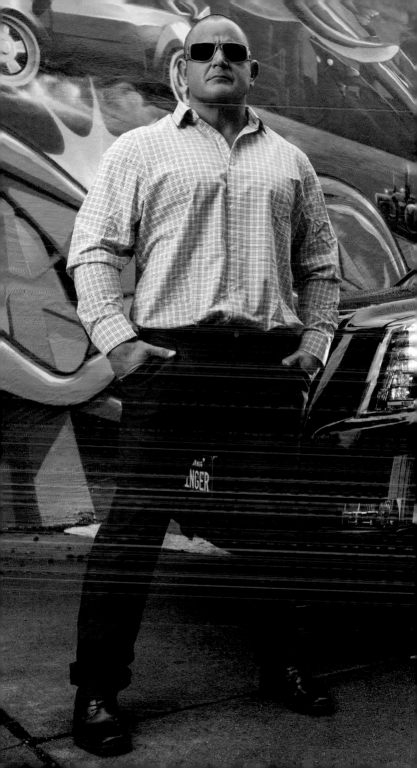

13. PERFORMANCE ENHANCING DIET – PED A TYPICAL DAY

Carbs before and after Training Session

If you're doing the PED diet, it looks just like the War on Carbs, except you'll add carbs before and after your workout. For me, carbs from something like rice or a sweet potato several hours before a training session work great. There has been new research showing that certain carbs, when heated and cooled, become a resistant starch. Resistant starches, such as sweet potatoes and sushi rice, are ideal for low-carb living. Post-workout, I have orange juice, or OJ + Gatorade to help replenish carbohydrates. Having my pre-workout carbohydrates come from food allows me to make an agreement with myself that I'm not going to eat any more food carbs the rest of the day. The only other source of carbs may come from my post-workout drink. Everyone's workout schedule is different, so you can experiment with this in whatever way you'd like. There's no reason to overthink it. There's research that refutes every single thing that has ever happened in the world. So play with it and see what gives you the best results.

TYPICAL DAY IF YOU'RE TRAINING SESSION IS AT 11 A.M.

9 a.m. – Gluten-free oatmeal or cream of rice + peanut butter and Walden Farms™ pancake syrup
11 a.m.* – Lifting
1 p.m. – Post workout – The "George Lockhart Cocktail" – 8 oz. of OJ with 8 oz. of Gatorade™ and 40-80mg of caffeine (I get the caffeine from Nuun energy tablets, which you can buy off of Amazon®)
3 p.m. – Steak
7 p.m. – Omelet with three eggs + cheddar cheese + bacon

*I advise always eating two hours before a training session so you don't feel like a hobo. You can sprinkle in the carbs up to four times a week or utilize them two times a week. You can also manipulate the amount of carbs you eat based on how lean you're getting. A leaner person might choose to add more carbs, where a fatter person may opt to have them less—experiment a little and find what works for you. And if you're stuck, don't be afraid to go against the grain and try something different. Sometimes all you need is to add some calories back into your diet or increase your fat intake.

By the way, on non-weight training days, you're still not going to consume any carbohydrates, fatass.

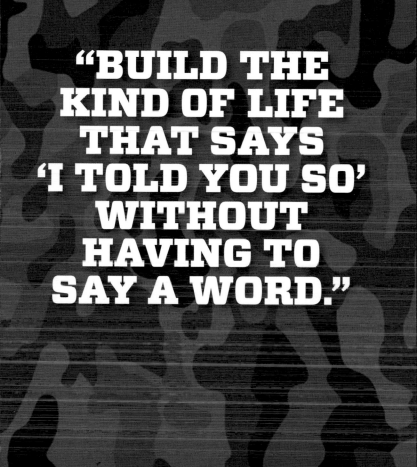

14. FASTING – A TYPICAL DAY

5 a.m. – Water
Noon – Water
2:30 p.m. – Water
5 p.m. – Water
9 p.m. – Water

REPEAT.

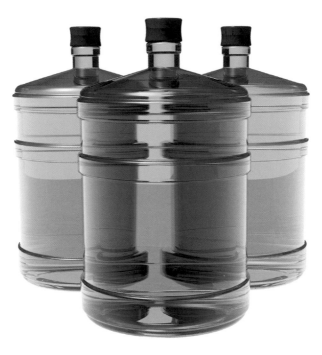

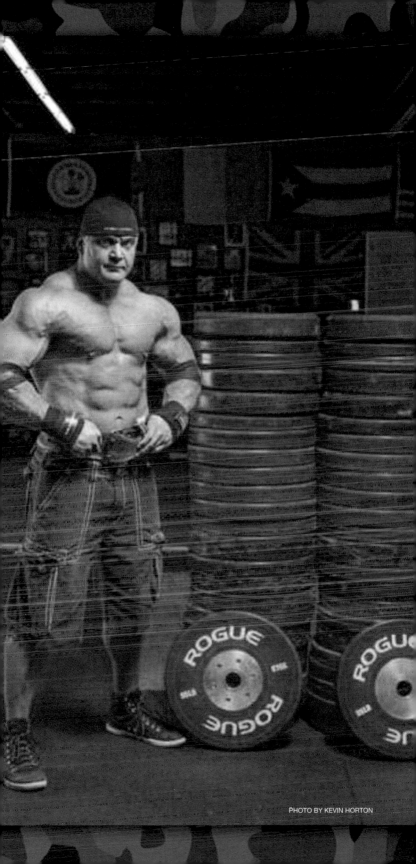

15. A TYPICAL WEEK WITH TRAINING

So you know you're not eating carbs, but what does your week look like? Here's what it looks like for me.

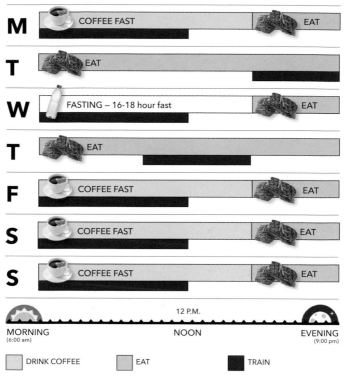

* Note this table indicates time frames. Your own schedule might vary.

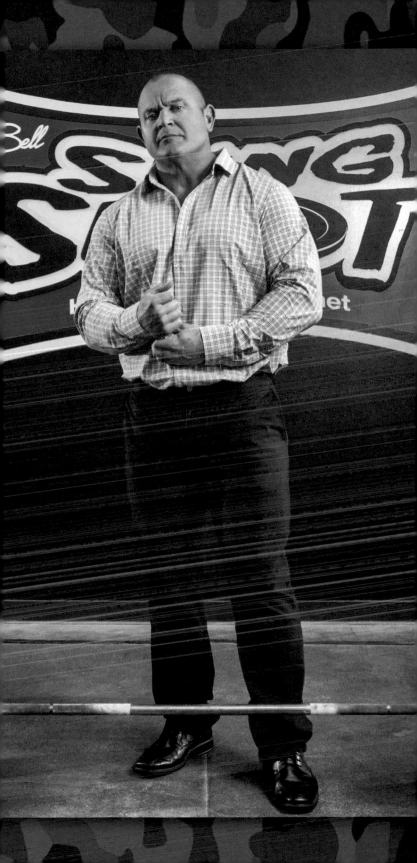

16. MARK'S SURVIVAL SNACKS

What's worked well for me is eating three meals a day. One smallish meal 2–3 hours before dinner, a full dinner, and then a snack before bed. Sometimes I end the day with something sweet, i.e. Keto Pro, Phat fudge, Keto Kookie, or something from Legendary Foods. Here's a list of my preferred snacks:

• Almonds
• Cashews
• Macadamia nuts
• Walnuts
• Duke's® Sausages
• Cheese
• Epic® Foods: most of their products are low in carbs
• Bone broth
• Hardboiled eggs
• Protein box at Starbucks®, just don't eat the fruit
• Phat Fudge
• Fat Bombs
• Walden Farms
• Real Good Pizza Company® – In a small personal-size pizza, there are only four carbohydrates, and they're gluten-free.
• Cured meats
• Natural peanut butter on a Keto Kookie
• Keto Pro® hot chocolate

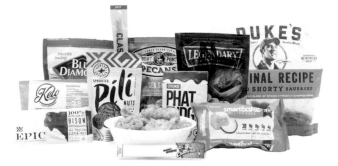

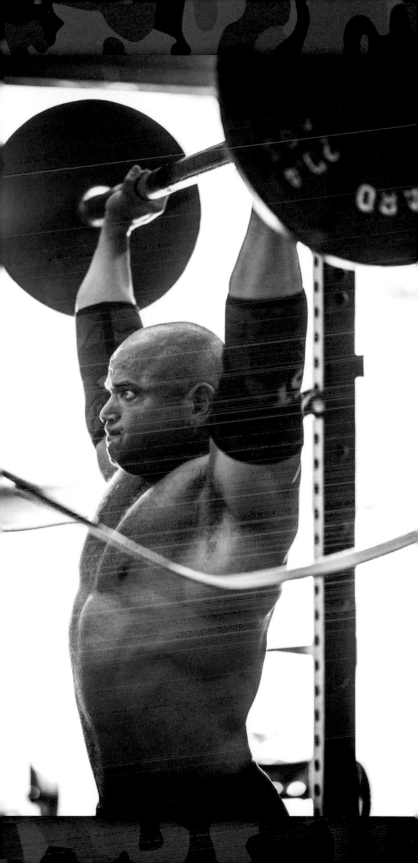

17. CHEAT MEALS

WHEN AND WHY

When you indulge in a cheat meal, you're technically off the War on Carbs. But there are a few things you can do before and after to mitigate the damage. Just because you're cheating and eating carbs doesn't mean you're completely kicked off the team. Your body may still be in ketosis.

Why cheat? Well why in the f*ck do you think? Carbs are delicious. However, I'd like to see everyone go 20 days or longer from the day you start without cheating. If you want a bigger goal, see if you can beat my record of 31 days.

The way we're going to keep your cheat meal from becoming a giant tsunami of carbs is by cheating within a cheat window. Once you commit to cheating, you only have 4-6 hours to do it. Once you're done with it, you're really done with it and it's in your rearview mirror. In that timeframe, you have two options. Option #1 is to limit the overall amount of carbohydrates that you eat and still have the potential of not being bumped out of ketosis. The amount of carbs associated with that is going to depend a lot from one person to the next. For myself, I would say it's under about 200 grams.

Option #2 is to be all in and just not even think about the consequences—just eat. With cheating on the War on Carbs, you will always need to do the following: pre-cheat prep and morning after damage control.

THE ART OF THE CHEAT MEAL –
FAST IN AND FAST OUT

As a pre-cheat prep, we're going to fast our way in and fast our way out. You're going to use a minimum of a 14-16 hour fast prior to your cheat, and then again to get back out of it. During that fast, you can use supplemental ketones and some exercise to help speed up the process.

A theory of Dan Duchaine's is that you could utilize a depletion workout to A) help you absorb the carbohydrates from cheating and B) help you deplete the carbohydrates on your way back onto the plan. I, too, believe in this method.

A depletion workout consists of a full-body circuit training workout with weights, and concludes with 6-8 20-second sprints on any piece of cardio equipment you'd like.

Please know, I'm not trying to promote a cheat. I'm not going to sit here and tell you that cheating or eating junk will speed up your metabolism. Junk food is junk food and in my opinion all it does is give us a break. Sometimes you need that, mentally. Although if you do break and do cheat, just call it what it is, and get right back on track the next day.

It's going to take dedication from all aspects of your life to get this plan to work the right way. To optimize all the benefits of this diet, you have to pay attention to your food, your training, and salt and water intake, while working really hard to change your already shitty sleeping habits. This is where a lot of the magic happens.

18. HYDRATION

You guys know that a ketogenic diet is absent of carbohydrates. And when you take out carbs, your insulin levels will be lower. When insulin is low, the kidneys excrete more water and sodium, which may lead to frequent urination and potential dehydration. Be smart and drink water. In addition to adding salt to some of your food and water throughout the day, you may want to supplement with other electrolytes, such as calcium, potassium and magnesium. To replenish potassium, you can focus on consuming foods that are high in potassium, such as avocados and green leafy vegetables like spinach.

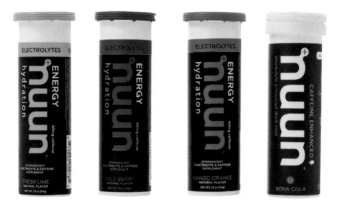

"REMEMBER THAT GUY THAT GAVE UP? NEITHER DOES ANYONE ELSE."

19. PROTEIN

In some cases, your protein may be too high and your fat may be too low.

Sometimes people's progress is halted by too much protein and too little fat. If we're keeping the fat on a level of 1g of fat per 1g of protein, there's nothing to worry about. To be on the safe side, maybe you want your ratio to be 1.25g of fat to 1g of protein. The only reason I looked into this is because people are paranoid about numbers and I had to give you answers. But it's nothing that I'm concerned with and it has not slowed me down. Again, consult with a doctor prior to starting this diet.

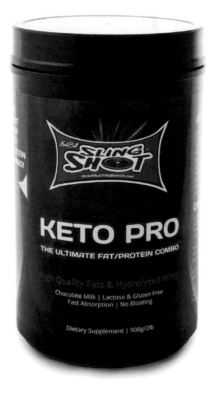

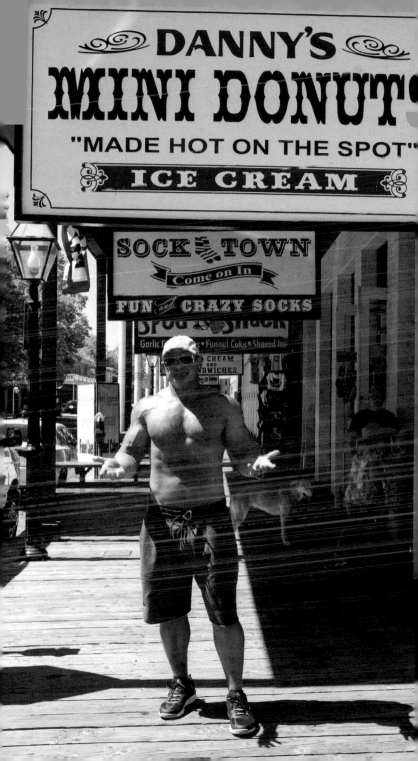

20. ALCOHOL

Come on, you can't have it all. Cutting out your alcohol completely will yield the best results. No question about it. Having some alcohol even once or twice a week will just slow down your progress — there's no other way to put it. However, drinking alcohol is fun. And who doesn't like to have fun here and there? I myself will have something to drink 1-2 times a week. I try to not go over three. Usually, I drink red wine because a typical glass of wine has four carbs. In my opinion, Dry Creek Farm Wines gives you the most bang for your buck for low carb/low sugar wine. Lastly, how many times have you had too much to drink and realized the next morning that you made a very bad decision? The same poor choices can happen with food. The chances of ending up knee-deep in pizza and ice cream when you're drunk are higher than when you're sober and in control.

There are better and worse alcohols for you. No-carb alcohols: Whiskey, rum, and vodka all have zero carbohydrates. But remember they still have calories.

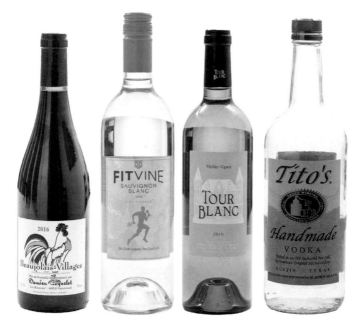

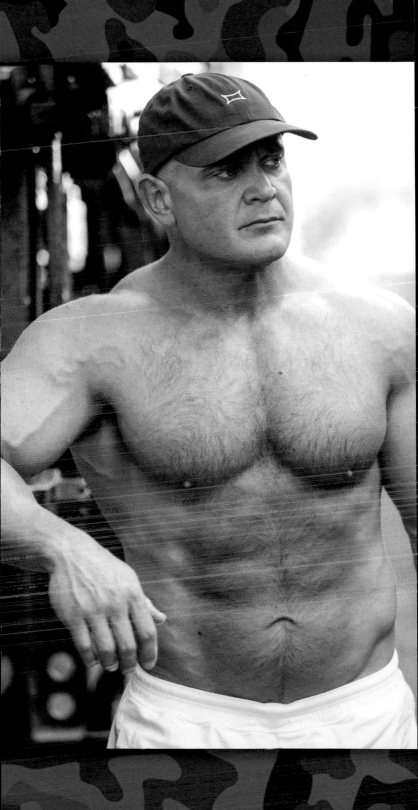

21. WHAT'S A FAT FAST?

If you feel like you're stuck, you can use a fat fast to help you out. I do this often to try to augment the percentages in my favor to keep the ketone production high. When using a fat fast, the food will be kept to a minimum. This is something you should do only for a short period of time. No longer than 2-3 days. This will help reset your body and can help you to get into ketosis faster. It might even help you get through a plateau or a sticking point.

EXAMPLES OF FOODS TO EAT DURING THE FAT FAST:

Bacon

Sausage

Avocado

Scrambled eggs: predominantly egg yolks with butter

As mentioned earlier, you can also use a coffee fast with MCT oil and butter as a fat fast like I do.

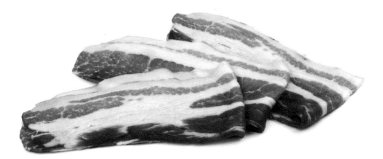

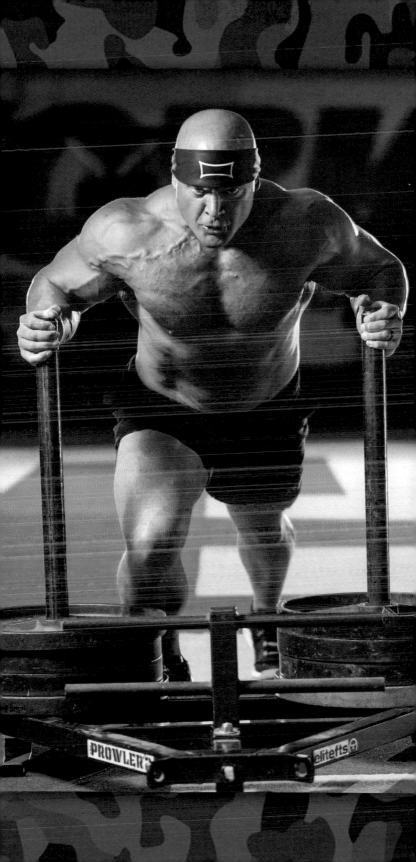

22. SLEEP

I used to wake up in the middle of the night and feel hungry. I would satisfy that hunger with junk, rarely something healthy. A lot of the time it was extra calories that I didn't need. It's just an onslaught of eating crappy food. I would eat peanut butter cups, ice cream, any junk I could find. And my wife would wake up the next day and see tons of candy wrappers in the garbage. I realized over time that I could train myself out of this. You can train yourself out of anything. I wasn't actually hungry, I just thought I was.

Your thoughts become your actions. So if you sit there and think about peanut butter cups, you're probably going to eat peanut butter cups. Your actions become your habits, so you have to train yourself out of bad actions before they become your habits. One leads to another.

You need to work on sleeping the same way you work on training.

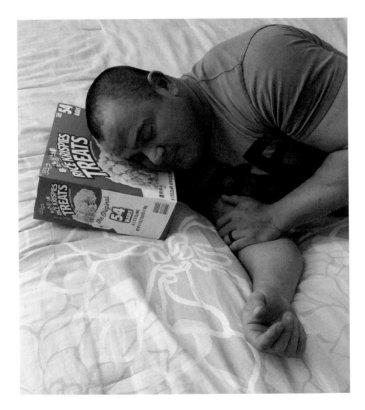

23. EXERCISE

I recognize that not everyone is super excited about exercise, but I feel that any exercise, especially lifting weights, is extremely beneficial to your overall health and body composition.

Exercises such as walking, and any form of steady-state cardiovascular training (elliptical, treadmill, exercise bikes), will help you burn calories for the duration of that training session – but they don't actually improve your metabolism. On the other hand, resistance training, liftin' some mothaf*ckin' weights, will help you increase muscle mass. And the more muscle mass that you have, the more calories you automatically burn even while you're just sitting or shitting. Plain facts: Weight training will help you improve your metabolism.

This book is designed to teach you about diet, so I'm not going to dive too much into lifting stuff.

I try to train every single day. Sometimes my training is simply just 30 minutes of walking, broken down into a couple 10-minute walks. I like to force myself to do things differently than everyone else. Many people get excited about the weekend and let themselves go. They drink, they party, they bullshit, and they don't end up sticking to the goals they have. That's why I've always trained on the weekend. The other reason I train on the weekend is because Super Training Gym is free, and I invite any and all of you to come check us out on any given Sunday.

Here's the chart again that details my training/fasting schedule.

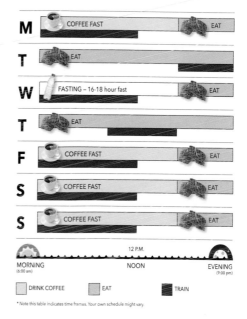

M — COFFEE FAST — EAT

T — EAT

W — FASTING – 16-18 hour fast — EAT

T — EAT

F — COFFEE FAST — EAT

S — COFFEE FAST — EAT

S — COFFEE FAST — EAT

12 P.M.

MORNING (6:00 am)   NOON   EVENING (9:00 pm)

DRINK COFFEE   EAT   TRAIN

* Note this table indicates time frames. Your own schedule might vary.

The other reason I train on the weekend is because Super Training Gym is open to visitors, and and I love meeting new people.

I like to end the week on a strong note. That's where I push my leg training, squats, deadlifts, etc. When it comes to strength training, there are a lot of resources out there. If you want to learn how to squat, bench, deadlift, etc. check out the Super Training YouTube channel at youtube.com/supertraining06. There's also a large variety of online coaches and apps you can use to help you with your fitness and strength goals.

Once a week we're using a full fast, which I've defined as being 16-18 hours and that's without consuming any calories. You can have coffee but you can't put anything in it. Tuesday and Thursday are both pretty intense training sessions, so on those days I just eat. Sometimes I may use a short fast, which would require that I start my eating between 9 and 11 a.m. Since I wake up at 5 a.m., that's several hours to wait before I eat.

Other days I have a coffee fast on the schedule. A coffee fast is drinking coffee with grass fed butter or ghee and MCT oil. That's it. Blend it up. You can have it hot or cold. Just a little recipe advice: if you put the MCT oil and butter in hot water first, it'll melt and be easier to blend into your coffee. When I blend up my coffee, I use the immersion blender or the Ninja. These are both good products that might help you out.

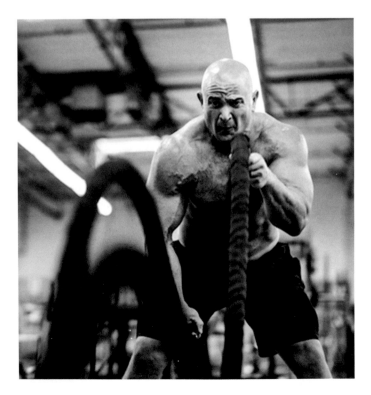

24. KETO PRO® HOT CHOCOLATE

INGREDIENTS:

- 1 scoop Keto Pro®
- Heavy whipping cream (watch it, fatty)
- Hot water
- Grass fed butter or coconut oil

INSTRUCTIONS:

- Use a blender to blend it up!

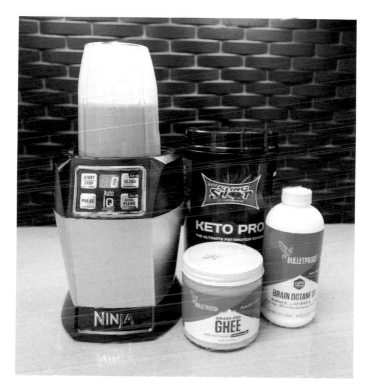

25. THE COFFEE FAST

I will define this as 12-14 hour fast, but you're drinking coffee with grass fed butter or ghee and MCT oil. The combination of the butter and MCT oil will give your body some fuel to run off of until it's time to eat. It can help stave off your hunger. This is a key element to not just losing weight but creating a new lifestyle. Because face it, most of us overeat. You can use the coffee fast as much as you want, but throughout this diet, I want you to ask yourself the question: How does this help and how does this hurt?

If you diet too hard and don't eat, you can screw yourself up. You could be restricting too much and not eating enough calories, which can also throw off our intent. In my opinion, the full fasting day that I have slated for once a week is plenty, but if you find you really enjoy it you can utilize it more. My advice to break the full-fasting day is to consume more than one meal to ease yourself into eating. For example, I have a small meal to break my fast about an hour or two before my main larger meal. This helps to better digest your food. I noticed that when I went straight into a regular meal after a fast, since I was really hungry, I ate too fast and too much. And that's a great way to blow up your stomach.

26. SUPPLEMENTS

Here is a list of supplements I take. You should always consult with a physician before beginning a supplement plan.

• Magnesium glycinate
• EPA-DHA 1000
• Digest-ALL
• Zinc
• Curcumin
• Zyflamend
• High-dose Electrolytes
• Magtein (Magnesium L-Threonate)
• Fenugreek Plus
• D3

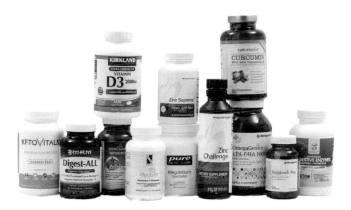

27. SUPPLEMENTAL KETONES

I often get asked questions about exogenous supplemental ketones. It is my belief that they do not necessarily help to stimulate fat loss, but they can help provide a little boost of energy and hydration. I have used them during my fasting day to help me with my energy levels. My personal feeling is that the word is still out on how effective they are. There's a huge difference between being in ketosis and registering high ketones on a ketone meter from drinking a supplement. I am a person who believes that ketosis must be earned .

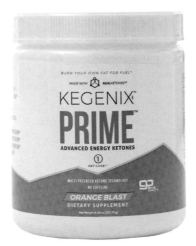

28. ADDICTION

The War on Carbs isn't necessarily about getting everyone into ketosis. It's about helping people abstain from overeating and addiction. This is a good opportunity for me to clear things up: I do not think carbs are bad. In fact, they are a great energy source to help you recover from workouts, hydrate muscles, enhance performance, preserve muscle mass, assist you in gaining lean muscle tissue, and a whole host of other things that are all positive. I have used them throughout my lifting career to lift weights that were heavier than I ever thought I could lift. But I also ended up heavier and fatter than I ever thought was possible. So, carbs aren't necessarily bad, but they are very easy to overeat. In my opinion, they are also highly addictive. If I could tell the world just a couple things about dieting, I would say don't eat fried food, don't overeat, and don't eat sugar. But if that was easy, then dieting in general wouldn't be a multi-billion-dollar industry.

Regarding my powerlifting career and working on weighing upwards of 330 lbs., it's not the fault of rice and berries and sweet potatoes that got me so fat. My diet promoted the overindulgence of carbs for the sake of performance. I was trying to stay big for lifting, and because I was trying to get as big as possible, I went too far into the rabbit hole.

I realize that we all have different taste buds, but get real with yourself. When was the last time you said, "I'm dying for spinach?" Or "I'm craving asparagus?" That's not what we do. We say, "I'd kill for some pizza." No one can argue with this. Something about carbs is just addictive, so it's easier to just stay away.

29. METABOLIC FLEXIBILITY

Metabolic flexibility is the ability to switch from one fuel source to the next. Your metabolism isn't stagnant. It shouldn't always sit in one place. It moves with your body fat percentages and muscularity. For example, if you do the War on Carbs for three months, you'll be leaner, your body fat percentage will be better, and therefore you will be able to move into switching up your diet a little or adding in carbs. Being deep into ketosis doesn't necessarily ensure that you're losing more body fat. But again, the whole point of being in ketosis is to have a manageable caloric intake while getting energy from ketones to supply your brain and body with the energy they need. Basically, you should be able to get results with variations of the diet. I suggest if you're a lardass, then you should be as strict as possible for as long as you can.

As you're making more progress with your body, you may have to continue to make changes to your diet to continue to make changes to your body. By not eating carbs for a long period of time, we may make ourselves susceptible to not being able to utilize them well. So maybe going in and out of the War on Carbs several months at a time might be a good idea. Any diet plan should have a start-up strategy and an exit strategy. You'll want to think about how you'll exit in and out of these diets. If you set a goal to lose 20lbs., it's not a great idea to lose the 20lbs. and not have an idea of what you'll do next. So before you even start, it's good to have an exit strategy. Because the worst thing you could do is lose 20 lbs. and gain 30 lbs.

30. LOW-CARB LIFE

Everyone has different levels of carb sensitivity. You could go low-carb and still have really positive results. In addition, you could be deep in ketosis and not necessarily burn a lot of fat or look significantly better. So sometimes, you may need to change it up by incorporating 50-100g of carbs per day. The benefit to taking in this amount of carbs per day would be to help preserve muscle mass or even gain muscle, whereas when you're on a strict keto diet it may be tougher to gain muscle mass due to the protein and carbohydrate restriction. In short, don't be afraid to mix shit up a little bit and experiment. That's what I've done over the years and it's always worked well for me.

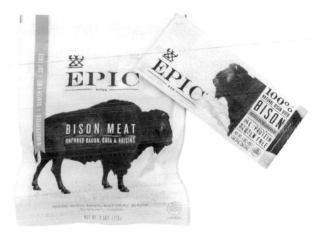

31. MORE KEYS TO SUCCESS

The things in this book are proven to be very effective. However, there are other very simple things that you can implement that can be extremely helpful to your diet or lifestyle.

1. TEN-MINUTE WALKS.
Fit a 10-minute walk into your day, and try to rack up 3-4 walks a week. Eventually get to two per day. These walks also aid in digestion and help with insulin sensitivity.

2. SLEEP.
Figure out a way to sleep eight hours a day and/or add in a 20-minute nap.

3. HYDRATION.
Water + salt. Consume 67% of your body weight in ounces of water every day. Ex: If you weigh 200 lbs., you should be drinking 134 ounces of water every day.

4. FOR EATING OUT.
Don't order appetizers. Don't eat the bread. Only eat half of what you order, and take the other half home. Drink lots of water with your meal. Eat slowly. Give yourself time to enjoy the meal and digest it.

5. DON'T BE DISTRACTED.
Eating in front of screens – TV screens, computer screens, and cell phone screens – can sometimes lead to digestive problems and not chewing properly. You want to sit down and concentrate on your food.

6. DOUBLE UP.
When you go somewhere that you like to eat, order the same meal to take home.

7. RECRUIT PEOPLE TO JOIN YOU ON YOUR WAR ON CARBS.
Recruit someone in your own house. That's what I do, and it's worked out great for me. That's right, everybody! Andee Bell has joined the War on Carbs, and she's a soldier just like you.

8. TELL PEOPLE WHAT YOU'RE DOING.
Put it out there in the universe. Stating it as a fact is even better. Instead of saying "I want to lose 10lbs." say "I'm going to lose 10lbs." Maybe even explain to people why. It's also something that you should put up on your social media.

9. INTERMITTENT FASTING.
Do 12-hour fasts and work them into being more substantial. Start out by doing 1-2 a week. Work your way up to doing 14-hour, 16-hour, 18-hour, and even 24-hour fasts. Fasting just means you're not going to eat any food. You can still drink water, coffee, or tea, but you're trying to keep the calories at zero.

10. PROTEIN SHAKES.

A protein shake can replace a meal and be something that stifles your hunger and delivers nutrition. I drink protein shakes before a meal or after a training session. By drinking a protein shake before a meal, it prevents me from overeating. It also destroys my sweet tooth. I can mix up my Sling Shot protein, or make my Keto Pro hot chocolate, and I won't have to think about peanut butter cups and cookies the rest of the night.

11. ADD FAT.

If you're having trouble getting enough fat in your diet, salad with dressing is an easy way to incorporate more oils.

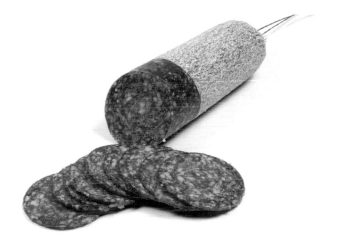

32. PEOPLE TO FOLLOW

Stan Efferding: Your life will just be better if you follow The Rhino. He earned a pro bodybuilding card while also in pursuit of world records in powerlifting. He is the embodiment of practicing what you preach, not just some skinny nerd who researches stuff . He's someone who is implementing stuff with himself and athletes around the world. @stanefferding

Mark Sisson: One glance at Mark Sisson's Instagram and you know the guy is the real deal, jacked at 64-years-old. He was a pivotal person in making people aware of how dangerous certain foods can be. He developed Primal Kitchen, providing a place for people to go to purchase health-conscious foods. More importantly, he's part of Dry Creek Farms, which sources keto-friendly wines from around the world. @marksdailyapple

Robb Wolf: He brings a science and research background to the table and in my opinion he's the one that put paleo-type diets on the map. @dasrobbwolf

John Kiefer: Years ago, John Kiefer made me aware of his diet Carb Nite, and that's initially what sent me down the path of losing weight and being healthier as professional powerlifter. @DHkiefer

Joe Rogan: You don't need me to explain who he is. Just follow him. No explanation needed. He's a badass. He's got the best podcast in the world. @joerogan

Andy Galpin: People talk a lot about topics they don't really know anything about. Andy actually knows because he is somebody who is actually in a lab, physically researching many of these topics. @drandygalpin

Dave Asprey: Some people feel that his ideas are outlandish. However, he has sold millions of cups of Bulletproof Coffee, despite people thinking that putting oil and butter in your coffee was off the wall. He made Bulletproof popular. @dave.aspreyHe made Bulletproof popular. @dave.asprey

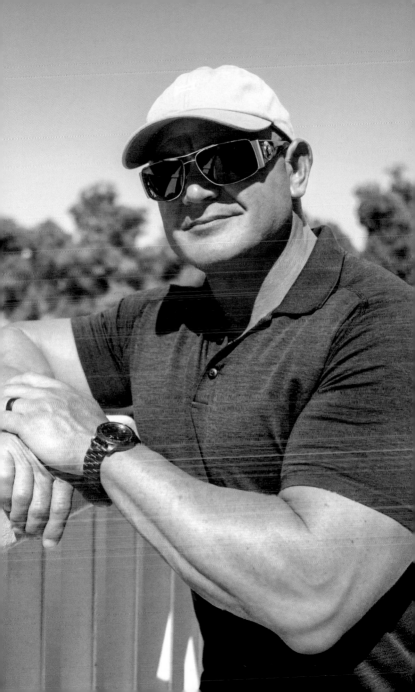

33. RECOMMENDED BOOKS

• The Bulletproof Diet, by Dave Asprey

• The Ketogenic Bible: The Authoritative Guide to Ketosis, by Dr. Jacob Wilson and Ryan Lowery, PhD

• Eat Bacon, Don't Jog, by Grant Petersen

• The Keto Diet: The Complete Guide to a High-Fat Diet, by Leanne Vogel

• The Keto Reset Diet, by Mark Sisson and Brad Kearns

• The Art and Science of Low Carbohydrate Living, by Jeff S. Volek and Stephen D. Phinney

• Fat Bombs, by Martina Slajerova

• The Ketogenic Cookbook, by Jimmy Moore

• Case Against Sugar, by Gary Taubes

• Obesity Code, by Jason Fong

• 25 Days, by Drew Logan and Myatt Murphy

• Wired to Eat, by Robb Wolf

34. RECOMMENDED WEBSITES

RULED.ME – Ruled.me is an amazing website loaded with information about keto recipes, keto snacks, and desserts, along with further descriptions of the keto diet, keto food lists, and more.

BULLETPROOF.COM – Dave Asprey's website is a good source of information and high-performance foods and supplements to help you along the way.

KETOCONNECT.NET – A hub for easy low-carb, gluten-free, and keto recipes, as well as tips on making the keto lifestyle more approachable.

MARKSDAILYAPPLE.COM – Mark Sisson's daily musings on health, nutrition, fitness, the health industry and the low-carb, paleo, Primal lifestyle.

KETOSUMMIT.COM – Free resources to help you lose weight, heal your body, solve underlying health issues, and look and feel better than ever with a low-carb, keto diet.

MARKBELLSLINGSHOT.COM – Your #1 source for all Sling Shot® products, including Keto Pro, to help you lead a healthy and fit lifestyle.

THEMARKBELL.COM – Any and everything Mark Bell! Including everything to do with Sling Shot®, POWER magazine, and the Super Training YouTube Channel.

THEPOWERMAGAZINE.COM – The home of the world's #1 powerlifting magazine.

35. Q & A

• **What do you eat on a keto diet?**

You eat meat and cheese and vegetables and nuts. For a more comprehensive list, refer to "The Diet" section of this book on page 16.

• **How do I get my body into ketosis?**

There are two main ways: one is to not eat carbs for an extended period of time. The other way is by fasting.

• **Is peanut butter good for keto?**

Yes. But make sure to get natural peanut butter with no sugar.

• **What does fat-adapted mean? Is it important to me?**

Fat-adapted means that you have adjusted to the diet and you've gone from just burning up some carbs to burning up some fat. Yes, being fat-adapted is important because once you get deeper in to the diet and are producing ketones, the ketones plus fat will be your energy source and it will keep your energy high.

• **What do you do if you're following this diet and you feel like shit?**

If you're following the diet and you feel like shit then you probably need to eat more fat. If you feel like you're doing that already, then you may just not be fat-adapted yet.

• **How many calories should I consume every day?**

I don't know. Every person is different, and I don't count my calories on this diet.

• **How much fat should I consume?**

Your fat intake should make up 70% or more if your overall calories. I personally achieve this level by augmenting my meals with various oils: Olive oil, coconut oil, MCT oil.

• **Is getting into ketosis the hardest part of the diet?**

Yes, it's the hardest part of the diet. It can take two days or two months — everyone's different. Most people will get there in a 14-day span. But for others, it could take several weeks or a full month. Troubleshooting and trying to figure out why you're not in ketosis can be a pain. Adjusting to eating such large amounts of fat can be a pain. To get to the 70-80% fat intake range can take a lot of trial and error and possibly many trips to the bathroom. My own experience with getting into ketosis was fairly simple: I didn't eat carbs, I added butter, MCT oil, olive oil, avocado oil, to meals and shakes and I exercised rigorously until I ended up in ketosis. But even with a strict adherence to the diet, and a tough training regimen, it still took me time to get into ketosis. In the beginning, when you're going through a funk period of waiting for your body to be fat-adapted, it can feel like suffering for some. Some symptoms that are associated with this low-carb limbo before you get into ketosis are fatigue, cramping, headaches, light headedness, and constipation, but once you actually get into ketosis, you're fat-adapted and your body is running off of fat, so those symptoms ease up.